Fit For Life!

NO DIETING
NO FOOD RESTRICTIONS
NO GRUELING WORKOUT SESSIONS

Watch the fat melt away as you unlock the secrets
to being fit for life! Yes, You Can!

T0105500

SUZANNE O'BRIEN
Personal Fitness Trainer

Library of Congress Control Number:		2008901148
ISBN:	Hardcover	978-1-4500-4569-8
	Softcover	978-1-4500-2738-0

To contact us:

takechargehealth@yahoo.com
www.takechargeofyourhealthtoday.com
845-337-0389

This book was printed in the United States of America.

To order additional copies of this book, contact:

Xlibris Corporation
1-888-795-4274
www.Xlibris.com
Orders@Xlibris.com

44430

Fit For Life!

Contents

To my son, Nicholas.

With Love Always,
Mom

Introduction

Are you tired of going on diets? Do you get frustrated when you don't keep up with an exercise schedule. Are you too exhausted after work to go to the gym? Well, if you answered yes, I can tell you that I have felt the same exact thing.

We go through "cycles" in our lives and our physical state reflects that. We can all remember a time when we had everything on target. We ate right, exercised regularly and got plenty of water. We felt great and our friends would comment on how good you looked. Then, for some reason we would slowly add some unhealthy food into the diet, maybe alcohol, skip a few workouts and all of a sudden we are back to our unhealthier self. The question is why do we ever go back? We were feeling so great, full of energy, looking fit, so why regress?

One of the biggest reasons that we go back is that we think of diets as temporary. How many times have you said "I'm going on a diet tomorrow!". Or "I'm going to lose 20lbs on such and such diet." The reality is that diets are only temporary. It's wonderful to lose 15lbs but then if you stop the habits you incorporated to lose it, guess what? It starts to come right back.

The only way to lose weight and keep it off is to make being fit a lifestyle. Incorporating activity and a balanced diet will keep you strong, slim, and full of energy. The key is to understand how your body works and find foods that taste great, and are also full of nutrients. Let me tell you, I used to eat fast food for most of my meals for a period of time in my life. I really did not know of healthy delicious food options. As a result I was lethargic and my body did not have lean strong muscles. Once you learn about food for fuel—as well as having it taste great—you are going to start to feel incredible. Now take that change and add in exercise and you will feel like a completely new person.

We've talked about nutrition and exercise, now let's take a moment and talk about being mentally fit. You might be saying mentally fit? What is that? Well you are right in asking that question. Most people don't think of being mentally fit. But, to be truely "fit for life!" All three components play a part.

The mind is the strongest part of your person. Do you have a positive attitude? Are you stressed most of the time? Are you experiencing feelings of depression? These are all very real emotions that most of us experience in todays demanding world. How often do you take five minutes out of your day to sit quietly and check out whats going on with you today? What needs do I have that I need to take care of? If you are like me, not often enough. Our lives are so fast paced that we are always going forward and forget to take time and enjoy the very moment you are in right now!

Fit for life!, encompasses the whole aspect of fitness. Get ready to make changes for a lifetime. Enjoy the ride!

Love,
Suzanne

Nutrition

Nutrition

Nutrition is a major component to health. What you eat affects your energy levels, well-being, and overall fitness. Eating habits can also be closely linked with certain diseases, disabling conditions, and other health problems. Of particular concern is the connection between lifetime nutritional habits and the risk of the major chronic diseases, including heart disease, cancer, stroke, and diabetes. On the more positive side, however, a well-planned diet in conjunction with a fitness program can help prevent such conditions and even reverse some of them.

Creating a diet plan to support maximum fitness and protect against disease is a two-part project. First, you have to know which nutrients are necessary and in what amounts. Second, you have to translate those requirements into a diet consisting of foods you like to eat that are both available and affordable. Once you have an idea of what constitutes a healthy diet for you, you may also have to make adjustments in your current diet to bring it into line with your goals.

Yes, food is delicious, but what is important for your health are the nutrients contained in those foods. Your body requires proteins, fats, carbohydrates, vitamins, minerals, and water—about forty-five essential nutrients. The word "essential" means that you must get these substances from food because your body is unable to manufacture them at all, or at least not fast enough to meet your physiological needs.

Nutrients are released into the body by the process of digestion, which breaks them down into compounds that the gastrointestinal tract can absorb and the body can use. In this form, the essential nutrients provide energy, build and maintain body tissues and regular body functions. There are six classes of essential nutrients—proteins, carbohydrates, fats, vitamins, minerals, and water.

Three of the six classes of nutrients supply energy: proteins, carbohydrates, and fats. Fats provide the most energy: nine calories per gram. Protein and carbohydrates each provide four calories per gram. Experts advise against high fat consumption, in part because fats provide so many calories. Given the typical American diet, most Americans do not need the extra calories to meet energy needs.

Meeting our energy needs is only one of the functions of food. All the nutrients perform other numerous vital functions. In terms of quantity, water is the most significant nutrient. The body is approximately 60 percent water and can survive only a few days without it. Vitamins and minerals are needed in much smaller quantities, but they are still vital.

Lets Eat!

Yes, food is delicious, but it is ultimately used to fuel the body. This does not mean we have to eat foods that are full of nutrients and taste like bark. On the contrary, there are so many fresh, natural foods that are full of amazing taste and texture—and yes—they are good for you too!

When you think of food I want you to think of balance. Balance is going to be your mantra for just about everything from now on. Loseing and gaining weight is a mathematical equation. How many calories go in versus how many calories go out! If the number of calories we take in is greater than the number of calories we take out we gain weight and vice versa. The key here is to become familiar with what nutrition value foods have. This might seem too difficult, but in reality foods are divided into 3 major categories. Yes, just 3, so it wont be that hard to master. Once you know how each nutrient gets used by the body, you can make educated balanced meal choices.

Proteins

Protein is an important component of muscle, bone, blood, enzymes, cell membranes, and some hormones. Protein can also provide energy at four calories per gram of protein weight. Proteins are composed of amino acids. Twenty common amino acids are found in food; nine of these are essential to an adult diet: histidine, isoleucine, leucine, lysine, methionine, phenylalanine, threonine, tryptophan, and aline. "Essential" means that they are required for normal health and growth but must be provided in the diet because the body manufactures them in insufficient quantities, if at all. The other eleven amino acids can be produced by the body as long as the necessary ingredients are supplied by foods.

Foods are rated as "complete" protein sources if they supply all nine essential amino acids in adequate amounts. They are classified as "incomplete" protein sources if they supply only some. Meat, fish, poultry, eggs, milk, cheese, and other foods from animal sources provide complete proteins. Incomplete proteins come from plant sources such as beans, peas, and nuts. These are good sources of most essential amino acids but are usually low in one or two. Different vegetable proteins are low in different amino acids, so combinations can provide complete proteins. Vegetarians who eat no foods from animal sources can obtain all essential amino acids by eating a wide variety of foods each day.

Fats

At nine calories per gram, fats (also known as lipids) are the most concentrated source of energy. The fats stored in your body represent usable energy, help insulate your body, and support and cushion your organs. Fats in the diet help your body absorb fat-soluble vitamins and add important flavor and texture to foods. During periods of rest and light activity, fats are the major body fuel. The nervous system, brain, and red blood cells are fueled by carbohydrates; but most of the rest of the body's organs are fueled by fats. Two fats—linoleic acid and alpha-linolenic acid—are essential to the diet. They are key regulators of such body functions as the maintenance of blood pressure and the progress of a healthy pregnancy.

Types and Sources of Fats

Most of the fats in food and in your body are in the form of triglycerides, which are composed of a glycerine molecule plus three fatty acids. A fatty acid is made up of a chain of carbon atoms with oxygen attached at the end and hydrogen atoms attached along the length of the chain. Fatty acids differ in the length of their carbon atom chains and in their degree of saturation (the number of hydrogens attached to the chain). If every available band from each carbon atom in a fatty acid chain is attached to a hydrogen atom, the fatty acid is said to be saturated. If not all the available bands are taken up by hydrogens, the carbon atoms in the chain will form double bands with each other. Such fatty acids are called unsaturated fats. If there is only one double band, they fatty acid is call monounsaturated. If there are two or more double bands, the fatty acid is called polyunsaturated. The essential fatty acids—linoleic and alpha-linolenic acds—are both polyunsaturated.

Food fats are often composed of both saturated and unsaturated fatty acids. The dominant type of fatty acid determines the fat's characteristics. Food fats containing large amounts of saturated fatty acids are usually solid at room temperature (these are called "fats"). They are generally found in animal products. The leading sources of saturated fat in the American diet are unprocessed animal flesh (hamburgers, steaks, roasts), whole milk, cheese, hot dogs, and lunch meats. Food fats containing large amounts of monounsaturated and polyunsaturated fatty acids are usually from plant sources and are liquid at room temperature (these are called "oils"). Olive, canola, and peanut oils contain mostly monounsaturated fatty acids. Sunflower, corn, and safflower oils contain mostly polyunsaturated fatty acids.

There are exceptions to these generalizations. When unsaturated vegetable oils undergo the process of hydrogenation, a mixture of saturated and unsaturated fatty acids is produced. Hydrogenation turns many of the double bands in unsaturated fatty acids into single bands, increasing the degree of saturation and producing a more solid fat from a liquid oil. Hydrogenation also produces trans fatty acids, unsaturated fatty acids with an atypical shape that affects their behavior during cooking and in the body. Food manufacturers use hydrogenation to increase the stability of an oil so it can be reused for deep frying—to improve the texture of certain foods, to keep oil from separating out of peanut butter, and to extend the shelf life of foods made with oil. Hydrogenation is the process used to transform a liquid oil into margarine or vegetable shortening.

Many baked and fried foods are prepared with hydrogenated vegetable oils, so they can be relatively high in saturated and trans fatty acids. Leading sources of trans fatty acids in the American diet are deep-fried; fast-foods such as french fries and fried chicken or fish; baked and snack foods such as cakes, cookies, pastries, doughnuts, and chips; and stick margarine. In general, the more solid a hydrogenated oil is, the more saturated and trans fats it contains. For example, stick margarine typically contains more saturated and trans fatty acids than tub or squeeze margarine does. Smaller amounts of trans fats are found naturally in meat and milk.

Hydrogenated vegetable oils are not the only plant fats that contain saturated fats. Palm and coconut oils, although derived from plants, are also highly saturated. On the other hand, fish oils, derived from an animal source, are rich in polyunsaturated fats.

Recommended Fat Intake

You need only about one tablespoon (fifteen grams) of vegetable oil per day incorporated into your diet to supply the essential fats. The average American diet supplies considerably more than this amount. In fact, fats make up about 33 percent of our caloric intake. (This is the equivalent of about seventy-five grams or five tablespoons of fat per day). Health experts recommended that we reduce our fat intake to 30 percent, but not less than 10 percent of total daily calories, with less than 10 percent coming from saturated fat.

Fats and Your Health

Different types of fats have very different effects on health. Many studies have examined the effects of dietary fat intake on blood cholesterol levels and the risk of heart disease. Saturated and trans fatty acids have been found to raise blood levels of low-density lipoprotein (LDL), or "bad" cholesterol, thereby increasing a person's risk of heart disease. Unsaturated fatty acids, on the other hand, lower LDL and may increase levels of high-density lipoprotein (HDL), or "good" cholesterol. To reduce the risk of heart disease, it is important to substitute unsaturated fats for saturated and trans fats.

Most Americans consume more saturated fat (11 percent of total calories) than trans fat (2-4 percent of total calories). The best way to reduce saturated fat in your diet is to lower your intake of meat and full-fat dairy products (whole milk, cream, butter, cheese, ice cream). To lower trans fats, decrease your intake of deep-fried foods and baked goods made with hydrogenated vegetable oils; use liquid oils rather than margarine. (Remember, the softer or more liquid a fat is, the less saturated and trans fat it is likely to contain.) Saturated fats are listed on the nutrition label of prepared foods. Trans fats are not, but you can check for the presence of hydrogenated oils on the ingredient list. If "partially hydrogenated" oils or fats or "vegetable shortening" appear near the top of the list, the product may be high in trans fats.

Research has indicated that certain forms of polyunsaturated fatty acids—known as omega-3 fatty acids and found in fish—may have a particularly positive effect on cardiovascular health. If the endmost double bands of a polyunsaturated fat occur, three carbons from the end of the fatty acid chain, an omega-3 form is produced. If the endmost double bands occur at the sixth carbon atom, an omega-6 form is produced. Most of the polyunsaturated fats currently consumed by Americans are omega-6 forms, primarily from corn oil and soybean oil. However, the consumption of omega-3 fatty acids in fish has been shown to reduce the tendency of blood to clot, to decrease inflammatory responses in the body, and to raise levels of HDL. Seven appears to lower the risk of heart disease in some people. Because of these benefits, nutritionists now recommend that Americans increase the proportion of omega-3 polyunsaturated fats in their deity by increasing their consumption of fish to two or more times a week. Mackerel, herring, salmon, sardines, anchovies, tuna, and trout are all good sources of omega-3 fatty acids.

Dietary fat can affect health in other ways. Diets high in fat are associated with an increased risk of certain forms of cancer, especially colon cancer. A high-fat diet can also make weight management more difficult. Because fat is a concentrated source of calories (nine calories per gram versus four calories per gram for protein and carbohydrate), a high-fat diet is often a high-calorie diet that can lead to weight gain. In addition, there is some evidence that calories from fat are more easily converted to body fat than calories from protein or carbohydrate.

Although more research is needed on the precise effects of different types and amounts of fat on overall health, a great deal of evidence points to the fact that most people benefit from lowering their overall fat intake to recommended levels and substituting unsaturated fats for saturated and trans fats.

Carbohydrates

Carbohydrates function primarily to supply energy to body cells. Some cells, such as those in the brain and other parts of the nervous system and in the blood, use only carbohydrates for fuel. During high-intensity exercise, muscles also get most of their energy from carbohydrates. When we don't eat enough carbohydrates to satisfy the needs of the brain and red blood cells, our bodies synthesize carbohydrates from proteins. In situations of extreme deprivation, when the diet lacks sufficient amounts of both carbohydrates and proteins, the body turns to its own proteins, resulting in severe muscle wasting. This rarely occurs, however, because the body's daily carbohydrate requirement is filled by just three or four slices of bread.

Simple and Complex Carbohydrates

Carbohydrates are classified into two groups: simple and complex. Simple carbohydrates contain only one—or two-sugar units in each molecule. A one-sugar carbohydrate is called a monosaccharide; a two-sugar carbohydrate, a disaccharide. Simple carbohydrates include sucrose (table sugar), fructose (fruit sugar, honey) maltose (malt sugar), and lactose (milk sugar). They provide much of the sweetness in foods. Simple carbohydrates are found naturally in fruits and milk and are added to soft drinks, fruit drinks, candy, and sweet desserts.

Starches and most types of dietary fiber are complex carbohydrates. They consist of chains of many sugar molecules and are called polysaccharides. Starches are found in a variety of plants, especially grains (wheat, rye, rice, oats, barley, legumes, and tubers—potatoes and yams). Most other vegetables contain a mix of starches and simple carbohydrates. Dietary fiber is found in fruits, vegetable and grains.

Many nutritionists also distinguish between refined (processed) and unrefined carbohydrates. The refinement of wheat flour, rice, and cereal grains transforms whole wheat flour to white flour, brown rice to white rice, and so on. Refined carbohydrates usually retain all the calories of their unrefined counterparts, but they tend to be much lower in fiber, vitamins, and minerals. In general, unrefined carbohydrates tend to take longer to chew and digest than refined ones. They also enter the bloodstream more slowly. This slower digestive pace tends to make people feel full sooner and for a longer period, lessening the chance that they will overeat and gain weight. It also helps keep blood sugar and insulin levels low, which may decrease the risk of diabetes and heart disease. For all these reasons, unrefined carbohydrates are recommended over those that have been refined.

During digestion in the mouth and small intestine, the body breaks down starches and disaccharides into monosaccharides, such as glucose, for absorption into the bloodstream. Once the glucose is absorbed, cells take it up and use it for energy. The liver and muscles also take up glucose and store it in the form of a starch called glycogen. The muscles use glycogen as fuel during endurance events or long workouts. Carbohydrates consumed in excess of the body's energy needs are changed into fat and stored. Whenever caloric intake exceeds caloric expenditure, fat storage can lead to weight gain. This is true whether the excess calories come from carbohydrates, proteins, or fats.

How Much Carbohydrate Should You Eat?

On the average, Americans consume over 250 grams of carbohydrates per day, well above the minimum of 50-100 grams of essential carbohydrate required by the body. However, health experts recommend that Americans increase their consumption of carbohydrates—particularly complex carbohydrates—to 55 percent of total daily calories.

Experts also recommend that Americans alter the proportion of simple and complex carbohydrates in the diet, lowering simple carbohydrate intake from 25 percent to 15 percent or less of total daily calories. To accomplish this change, reduce your intake of foods like candy, sweet desserts, soft drinks, and sweetened fruit drinks, which are high in simple sugars but low in other nutrients. The bulk of the simple carbohydrates in your diet should come from fruits, which are excellent sources of vitamins and minerals, and milk, which is high in protein and calcium. Instead of prepared foods high in added sugars, choose a variety of foods rich in complex, unrefined carbohydrates.

Fiber

Dietary fiber consists of carbohydrate plant substances that are difficult or impossible for humans to digest. Instead, fiber passes through the intestinal tract and provides bulk for feces in the large intestine, which in turn facilitates elimination. In the large intestine, some types of fiber are broken down by bacteria into acids and gases, which explain why consuming too much fiber can lead to intestinal gas. Because humans cannot digest dietary fiber, fiber is not a source of carbohydrate in the diet. However, the consumption of dietary fiber is necessary for good health.

Nutritionists classify dietary fiber as soluble or insoluble. Soluble fiber slows the body's absorption of glucose and binds cholesterol-containing compounds in the intestine, lowering blood cholesterol levels and reducing the risk of cardiovascular disease. Insoluble fiber binds water, making the feces bulkier and softer so they pass more easily and quickly through the intestines.

Both kinds of fiber contribute to disease prevention. A diet high in soluble fiber can help people manage diabetes and high blood cholesterol levels. A diet high in insoluble fiber can help prevent a variety of health problems, including constipation, hemorrhoids, and diverticulitis (a painful condition in which abnormal pouches form and become inflamed in the wall of the large intestine. Some studies have linked high levels of insoluble fiber in the diet with a decreased incidence of colon and rectal cancer; conversely, a low-fiber diet may increase the risk of colon cancer. There is even some evidence that high levels of insoluble fiber can suppress and reverse precancerous changes that can lead to colon and rectal cancer.

All plant foods contain some dietary fiber; but fruits, legumes, oats (especially oat bran), barley, and psyllium (found in some laxatives) are particularly rich in it. Wheat (especially wheat bran), cereals, grains, and vegetables are all good sources of insoluble fiber. However, the processing of packaged foods can remove fiber, so it's important to depend on fresh fruits and vegetables and foods made from whole (unrefined) grains as sources of dietary fiber.

Most experts believe the average person would benefit from an increase in daily fiber intake. Currently, most people consume about 15 grams of fiber a day, whereas the recommended daily amount is 20-35 grams of food fiber—not from supplements, which should be taken only under medical supervision. However, too much fiber—more than 40-60 grams a day—can cause health problems such as overlarge stools or the malabsorption of important minerals. In fiber intake, as in all aspects of nutrition, balance and moderation are key principles.

To increase the amount of fiber in your diet, try the following:

- Chose whole grain bread instead of white bread, brown rice instead of white rice, and whole wheat pasta instead of regular pasta.
- Select high-fiber breakfast cereals. Look for breads, crackers, and cereals that list a whole grain first in the ingredient list: whole wheat flour, whole grain oats, and whole grain rice are whole grains. White flour is not.
- Eat whole fruits rather than drinking fruit juice. Top cereals, yogurts, and desserts with berries, apple slices, or other fruits.
- Include beans in soups and salads. Prepare salads that combine raw vegetables with pasta, rice, or beans.
- Substitute bean dip for cheese-based or sour cream-based dips or spreads. Use raw vegetables rather than chips for dipping.

Vitamins

Vitamins are organic (carbon-containing) substances required in very small amounts to promote specific chemical reactions within living cells. Humans need thirteen vitamins. Four are fat soluble (A, D, E, and K); and nine are water soluble (C); and the eight B-complex vitamins: thiamin, riboflavin, niacin, vitamin B-6, folate, vitamin B-12, biotin, and pantothenic acid. Solubility affects how a vitamin is absorbed, transported, and stored in the body. The water-soluble vitamins are absorbed directly into the bloodstream where they travel freely. Excess water-soluble vitamins are detected by the kidneys and excreted in urine. Fat-soluble vitamins require a more complex digestive process; they are usually carried in the blood by special proteins and are stored in the body in fat tissues rather than excreted.

Vitamins and Their Functions

Vitamins help chemical reactions take place. They provide no energy to the body directly but help unleash the energy stored in carbohydrates, proteins, and fats. Vitamins are critical in the production of red blood cells and the maintenance of the nervous, skeletal, and immune systems. Some vitamins also form substances that act as antioxidants, which help preserve healthy cells in the body. Key vitamin antioxidants include vitamin E, vitamin C, and the vitamin A derivative beta-carotene.

Sources of Vitamins

The human body does not manufacture most of the vitamins it requires and must obtain them from foods. Vitamins are abundant in fruits, vegetables, and grains. In addition, many processed foods, such as flour and breakfast cereals, are enriched with certain vitamins during the manufacturing process. On the other hand, both vitamins and minerals can be lost or destroyed during the storage and cooking of foods.

A few vitamins are made in certain parts of the body: the skin makes vitamin D when it is exposed to sunlight, and intestinal bacteria make biotin and vitamin K.

Minerals

Minerals are inorganic (noncarbon-containing) compounds you need in relatively small amounts to help regulate body functions, aid in the growth and maintenance of body tissues, and help release energy. There are about seventeen essential minerals. The major minerals—those that the body needs in amounts exceeding one hundred milligrams—include calcium, phosphorus, magnesium, sodium, potassium, and chloride. The essential trace minerals—those that you need in minute amounts—include copper, fluoride, iodine, iron, selenium, and zinc.

Characteristic symptoms develop if an essential mineral is consumed in a quantity too small or too large for good health. The minerals most commonly lacking in the American diet are iron, calcium, zinc, and magnesium. Lean meats are rich in iron and zinc, while low-fat or nonfat dairy products are excellent sources for calcium. Plant foods are good sources of magnesium. Iron-deficiency anemia is a problem in some age groups, and researchers agree that poor calcium intakes are laying the foundation for future osteoporosis, especially in women.

Drink Up! (Water)

Water is the major component in both foods and the human body: You are composed of about 60 percent water. Your need for other nutrients, in terms of weight, is much less than your need for water. You can live up to fifty days without food, but only a few days without water.

Water is distributed all over the body, among lean and other tissues and in urine and other body fluids. Water is used in the digestion and absorption of food and is the medium in which most of the chemical reactions take place within the body. Some water-based fluids like blood transport substances around the body, while other fluids serve as lubricants or cushions. Water also helps regulate body temperature.

Water is contained in almost all foods, particularly in liquids, fruits, and vegetables. The foods are fluids you consume provide 80-90 percent of your daily water intake; the remainder is generated through metabolism. You lose water each day in urine, feces, and sweat and through evaporation in your lungs. To maintain a balance between water consumed and water lost, you need to take in about one milliliter of water for each calorie you burn—about two liters (or eight cups) of fluid per day, more if you live in a hot climate or engage in vigorous exercise.

Thirst is one of the body's first signs of dehydration that we can actually recognize. However, by the time we are actually thirsty, our cells have been needing fluid for quite some time. So drink before you are thirsty. Keep a record of how much water you drink a day. Remember, you need eight, eight-ounce glasses—so drink up!

Amazing Antioxidants

When the body uses oxygen or breaks down certain fats as a normal part of metabolism, it gives rise to substances called free radicals. Environmental factors such as cigarette smoke, exhaust fumes, radiation, excessive sunlight, certain drugs, and stress can increase free radical production. A free radical is a chemically unstable molecule that is missing an electron; it will react with any molecule it encounters from which it can take an electron. In their search for electrons, free radicals react with fats, proteins, and DNA, damaging cell membranes and mutating genes. Because of this, free radicals have been implicated in aging, cancer, cardiovascular disease, and degenerative diseases like arthritis.

Antioxidants found in foods can help rid the body of free radicals, thereby protecting cells. Antioxidants react with free radicals and donate electrons, rendering them harmless. Some antioxidants—such as vitamin C, vitamin E, and selenium—are also essential nutrients. Others, such as flavonoids found in citrus fruits, are not. Obtaining a regular intake of these nutrients is vital for maintaining health. Many fruits and vegetables are rich in antioxidants.

Fantastic Phytochemicals

Antioxidants are a particular type of phytochemical, a substance found in plant foods that may help prevent chronic disease. Researchers have just begun to identify and study all the different compounds found in foods, and many preliminary findings are promising. For example, certain proteins found in soy foods may help lower cholesterol levels. Sulforaphane, a compound isolated from broccoli and other cruciferous vegetables, may render some carcinogenic compounds harmless. Allyl sulfides, a group of chemicals found in garlic and onions, appear to boost the activity of cancer-fighting immune cells. Further research on phytochemicals may extend the role of nutrition to the prevention and treatment of many chronic diseases.

If you want to increase your intake of phytochemicals, it is best to obtain them by eating a variety of fruits and vegetables rather than relying on supplements. It is likely that their health benefits are the result of chemical substances working in combination. Like many vitamins and minerals, isolated phytochemicals may be harmful if taken in high doses, so eat a variety of foods and enjoy all the benefits that phytochemicals have to offer.

Express Fit Nutrition Tips

Remember that our stomach expands. If you make two fists with your hands, put them side by side. This is approximately the size of your stomach. The key is to eat until you are not hungry anymore.

- Do not eat till you are full, this will stretch the stomach, and as a result it will take a large amount of food to make you feel satisfied for your next meal, due to the expansion. This becomes a viscious cycle and now you have much more calorie intake than output remember *balance.*
- Never eat anything *White.* Everything white is refined high glucose food with no fiber or nutrient content. These foods are empty calories that will cause a spike in blood sugar only to have you craving more food when the sugar goes down.
- Eat "clean" a good rule of thumb is to have nothing Processed. Eat a staple of fresh fruits and vegetables with preferably organic meats. Protein and complex carbohydrates are your main food groups to choose from.

Water Water Water—I know I said it alot, but I cannot stress enough the importance of water. Our bodies are composed of 60% of it. We cannot metabolize fat with out enough water so cheers! 8 8oz glasses a day please. PS your skin will be radiant too!

Let's Get Moving!

Your Thirty-Day Weight Loss and Fitness Program

Congratulations! You did it!

You took the first step that will change the rest of your life. My thirty-day weight loss and fitness program will empower you to have more energy and enthusiasm for life on an everyday basis. On our journey together, you will cleanse your body of toxins; and the exercise segment will help boost your metabolism to burn fat, lose weight, and give you more energy to live your life and make you feel happier every day. There's a saying—and it is very true—"Look better, feel better, do better!"

And there's more! As you read in the first section of the book, diet and exercise play a major role in the prevention of many debilitating diseases. Not only will you look great and feel incredible, but you will be helping yourself live a long and healthy life. What could be better?

In 1966, the U.S. Surgeon General's Report on physical activity and health was a call to encourage more Americans to become active. The report states that by becoming moderately active, Americans can lower their risk of premature death and the development of chronic illnesses such as heart disease, hypertension, and diabetes. (I would also like to add osteoporosis—brittle bones.) Among its major findings were the following points:

- People who are usually inactive can improve their health and well-being by becoming even *moderately* active on a regular basis.
- Physical activity does not need to be strenuous to achieve health benefits.
- Enhanced fitness and physiological changes occur when the amount (frequency, intensity, and duration) of the activity is increased.

Guidelines from the Surgeon General's Report include the following:

- Acquire thirty minutes of moderate activity on most, if not all, days of the week.
- A moderate amount of physical activity uses approximately 150 calories per day or one thousand calories per week.

It has been medically proven that exercise and nutrition are your best defense against becoming chronically ill.

The plan is thirty days because it takes thirty days for your subconscious mind to engrave a new habit into its system. Most of the reasons why we do not eat right, drink enough water, and exercise are the results of bad habits. Your subconscious mind is programmed to do these bad habits. So it will take a conscious effort to undo them and reprogram your mind with positive lifestyle changes.

I have mapped out your next thirty days with healthy eating suggestions, exercises, and motivational tips. All you need to do is follow the daily "recipe for success," and your subconscious mind will kick in and make these new habits your own.

In today's world, women and men wear many different hats. We are mothers and fathers, employees, wives and husbands. The stress level is high, and that is why it is so important to take time for you. This plan is yours. Give it to yourself, because you can't take care of anyone else unless you take good care of yourself first! Having more energy for life, looking great, reducing stress, and preventing disease are what this plan will do.

Disease is the result of a part of the body not getting the nutrients it needs. One of the best ways to make sure that your body is fully functioning is to aerobically exercise. When you are exercising aerobically, you are increasing your heart rate. The heart muscle is exercised to beat faster so that it can pump blood to every cell in the body and give it the oxygen it needs to perform respiration on a cellular level. At the same time, the lungs are breathing in fresh oxygen and ridding the body of carbon dioxide. The fresh oxygen is carried by the blood throughout the entire body. The result: disease prevention.

There are so many parts to the human body. If a person does not exercise and eats a diet of foods high in saturated fats, the circulatory system (blood vessels) are moving at a sluggish rate and may have blockages in the vessels (fat deposits). If this occurs, areas in your body may not be getting all the nutrients they need to function properly. Each and every cell in your body carries on cellular respiration. Each cell has a life of its own. It needs food and water, and it needs to rid itself of waste. If it does not get the energy it needs and waste builds up, it will start to die or mutate into an abnormal cell, and disease will occur.

Aerobic exercise will prevent this from happening. By exercising the heart thirty minutes a day, five times a week, every cell in your body will receive fresh, oxygenated blood and will release waste from it that will travel through the bloodstream and will be eliminated from the body through your gastrointestinal system, sweat in the skin, or lungs as carbon dioxide. The result is that you are ridding your body of toxins and ensuring that each cell in your body is functioning at its optimum level—and you will feel fantastic!

Let's Get Started!

Every exercise program includes three components: cardiorespiratory fitness, strength training and flexibility.

Cardiorespiratory Fitness

Cardiorespiratory fitness uses the aerobic energy system. Aerobic means air. It is defined as the ability to perform repetitive, moderate-to-high-intensity, large-muscle movements for a prolonged period of time using oxygen. Cardiorespiratory exercise is the most efficient way to reduce weight because it uses fat for fuel. There are also several other benefits to this form of exercise, including:

- stronger heart
- lowered blood pressure
- increased high-density lipoprotein
- stronger bones
- improved sleep
- decreased body fat
- increased ability to perform work with less fatigue
- increased cardiac output
- improved cholesterol ratio
- decreased stress
- decreased depression
- improved immune system
- improved glucose tolerance and insulin sensitivity
- improved quality of life
- decreased resting heart rate
- increase metabolism
- increased endurance, stamina, and energy
- increased ability to metabolize fat

To be effective, aerobic workouts depend on three variables: frequency, intensity, and duration.

Frequency

A frequency of three to five days per week is recommended. If you are trying to lose those extra pounds, four to five days a week are better than three. A beginner should start by doing three days a week, and if that person has not exercised in a long time and is "deconditioned," they can do several small bouts of ten-minute segments.

Intensity

Intensity is a very important component to aerobic exercise. The total amount of work performed is one of the most significant factors in improving cardiorespiratory fitness. Low-to-moderate-intensity training programs with longer durations are recommended for most adults. This decreases the risk of injury and increases adherence (sticking with it).

How to Figure Out the Right Intensity for You

There are two methods that we will use to find your correct intensity of aerobic exercise. The first is the HR method. This method is very simple and is used in most health clubs.

Take the number 220 and subtract your age. That will give you your estimated maximal heart rate. A person needs to work at an intensity of 50-85 percent of their maximal heart rate to achieve the benefits of cardiorespiratory training.

Example 1

1. 220 - age = estimated maximal heart rate
2. Estimated maximal heart rate x percentage (e.g. 70 percent) = target heart rate.

To take your heart rate, palpate the radial artery at your wrist with your forefinger and index finger. Once you find your pulse, count the number of beats for one full minute (or you can count the number of beats for ten seconds and multiply by six). This will give you your heart rate.

Example 2

Let's say you are forty years old and want to work at an intensity of 75 percent of heart rate maximum:

1. 220 - 40 = 180 (estimated heart rate maximum)
2. 180 x 0.75 = 135 BPM (beats per minute)

Immediately after aerobically exercising, take your pulse for one minute, either by counting beats for a full minute or by taking your pulse for ten seconds and multiplying it by six. Your heart rate should be at 135 to be working at an intensity of 75 percent.

Fit For Life!

To make it easy, you can use the following target heart rate training zone chart. In this chart, you see two numbers divided by a slash in each of the percentage columns. The first number is for the working heart rate. The second number is the number of heartbeats to count for ten seconds. You can use the second number if you don't want to do the multiplication to find your working heart rate.

TARGET HEART RATE TRAINING ZONE CHART			
Age	80%	70%	60%
15	164/27	144/24	123/21
16	163/27	143/24	122/21
17	162/27	142/24	122/21
18	162/27	141/24	121/20
19	161/27	141/24	121/20
20	160/27	140/23	120/20
21	159/27	139/23	119/20
22	158/26	139/23	119/20
23	158/26	138/23	118/20
24	157/26	137/23	118/20
25	156/26	137/23	117/20
26	155/26	136/23	116/19
27	154/26	135/23	116/19
28	154/26	134/22	115/19
29	153/26	134/22	115/19
30	152/25	133/22	114/19
31	151/25	132/22	113/19
32	150/25	132/22	113/19
33	150/25	131/22	112/19
34	149/25	130/22	119/19
35	148/25	130/22	119/19
36	147/25	129/22	110/18
37	146/24	128/21	110/18
38	146/24	127/21	109/18
39	145/24	127/21	109/18
40	144/24	126/21	108/18
41	143/24	125/21	107/18
42	142/24	124/41	107/18
43	142/24	124/21	106/18
44	141/24	123/21	106/18
45	140/23	123/21	105/18
46	139/23	122/20	104/17
47	138/23	121/20	104/17
48	138/23	120/20	103/17

49	137/23	120/20	103/17
50	136/23	119/20	102/17
51	135/23	118/20	101/17
52	134/22	118/20	101/17
53	134/22	117/20	100/17
54	133/22	116/19	100/17
55	132/22	116/19	99/17
56	131/22	115/19	98/16
57	130/22	114/19	98/16
58	130/22	113/19	97/16
59	129/22	113/19	97/16
60	128/21	112/19	93/16
61	127/21	111/19	95/16
62	126/21	111/19	95/16
63	126/21	110/18	94/16
64	125/21	109/18	94/16
65	124/21	108/18	93/16
66	123/21	108/18	92/15
67	122/20	107/18	92/15
68	122/20	106/18	91/15
69	121/20	106/18	91/15
70	120/20	105/18	90/15
71	119/20	104/17	89/15
72	118/20	104/17	89/15
73	118/20	103/17	88/15
74	117/20	102/17	88/15
75	116/19	102/17	87/15
76	115/19	101/17	86/14
77	114/19	100/17	86/14
78	114/19	99/17	85/14

Borg RPE Scale

Another way of assessing cardiorespiratory endurance is the rate of perceived exertion (RPE) method. It is valuable for determining intensity for several reasons, including helping clients to "listen to their bodies" and to anticipate approaching fatigue. The rate of perceived exertion can be used in conjunction with the heart rate method.

Using the original Borg scale of RPE, a rate of 12-13 approximates 50 percent of heart rate maximum and a rate of 16 approximates 85 percent of heart rate maximum. Therefore, it is recommended that you exercise within an RPE range of 12-16, meaning that the intensity feels somewhat hard to hard.

	RPE (BORG) SCALE	
	6	No exertion at all
	7	Very, very light
	8	
	9	Very light
	10	
50%	11	Light
	12	
	13	Somewhat hard
	14	
	15	Hard
85%	16	
	17	Very hard
	18	
	19	Extremely hard
	20	Maximal exertion

Duration (Time)

It is recommended that a person exercise for twenty to sixty minutes continuously doing aerobic activity. This does not include warm-up and cooldown. Duration is inversely related to intensity: The lower the intensity, the longer the duration may be. For very de-conditioned people, several low-intensity, short-duration, ten-minute sessions may be more suitable.

Some examples of aerobic exercises are power walking, jogging, aerobic dancing, spinning, stair stepping, stationary cycling, indoor rowing, indoor cross-country skiing, jumping rope, outdoor cycling, outdoor rowing, swimming, and recreational sports.

How to Find Out How Cardiovascularly Fit You Are

It is very important to assess your current level of aerobic fitness so that you don't overdo or underdo your aerobic exercises. The step test is an easy way to calculate your cardiovascular fitness.

What You Need:	A box or a step
	A stopwatch or a clock with a second hand
	Someone to help you time the test
What to Do:	Start stepping up and down in a rhythmic motion on and off the step for a full three minutes. As soon as you're done, find your pulse and record the number of beats for one full

41

minute. You can also count your beats for ten seconds and multiply the number by six to get the total number of beats per minute. Check your fitness level in the following charts:

Norms for the Three-Minute Step Test (Men)			
	Age		
Fitness Category	18-25	26-35	36-45
Excellent	<79	<81	<83
Good	79-89	81-89	83-96
Above Average	90-99	90-99	97-103
Average	100-105	100-107	104-112
Below Average	106-116	108-117	113-119
Poor	117-128	118-128	120-130
Very Poor	>128	>128	>130
	Age		
Fitness Category	46-55	56-65	65+
Excellent	<87	<86	<88
Good	87-97	86-97	88-96
Above Average	98-105	98-103	97-103
Average	106-116	104-112	104-113
Below Average	117-122	113-120	114-120
Poor	123-132	121-129	121-130
Very Poor	>132	>129	>130

Norms for the Three-Minute Step Test (Women)			
	Age		
Fitness Category	18-25	26-35	36-45
Excellent	<85	<88	<90
Good	85-98	88-99	90-102
Above Average	99-108	100-111	103-110
Average	109-117	112-119	111-118
Below Average	118-126	120-126	119-128
Poor	127-140	127-138	129-140
Very Poor	>140	>138	>140
	Age		
Fitness Category	46-55	56-65	65+
Excellent	<94	<95	<90
Good	94-104	95-104	90-102
Above Average	105-115	105-112	103-115
Average	116-120	113-118	116-122
Below Average	121-126	119-128	123-128
Poor	127-135	129-139	129-134
Very Poor	>135	>139	>134

Muscular Strength and Endurance

The muscles in your body make up over 40 percent of your total body mass. Due to the large percentage of space they take up, they are responsible for a major portion of the energy reactions that take place in your body.

Metabolism is also known as energy consumption and is what is used to burn the calories we eat. Our metabolism will also burn stored energy in our bodies (fat) if it needs energy to do work and if it is not readily available. Muscle mass burns five times more calories than fat. The more muscle mass your body has, the higher your metabolism or energy burning capacity will be.

Several benefits of enhanced muscular strength and endurance:

- enhanced self-image
- injury prevention
- improved body composition
- improved performance of physical activities
- improved muscle and bone health with aging

Enhanced Self-Image

Weight training leads to an enhanced self-image by providing stronger, firmer-looking muscles and a toned, healthy-looking body. Men tend to build larger, stronger, more shapely muscles. Women tend to lose inches, increase strength, and develop greater muscle definition.

Because weight training provides measurable objectives (pounds lifted, repetitions accomplished), a person can easily recognize improved performance, leading to greater self-confidence.

Injury Prevention

Increased muscle strength provides protection against injury because it helps people maintain good posture and appropriate body mechanics when carrying out everyday activities like walking, lifting, and carrying. Strong muscles in the abdomen, hips, low back, and legs support the back in proper alignment and help prevent low-back pain, which afflicts over 85 percent of all Americans at some time in their lives. Training for muscular strength also makes the tendons, ligaments, and joint surfaces stronger and less susceptible to injury.

Improved Body Composition

Healthy body composition means that the body has a high proportion of fat-free mass (primarily composed of muscle) and a relatively small proportion of fat. Strength training improves body composition by increasing muscle mass, thereby tipping the body composition ratio toward fat-free mass and away from fat.

Building muscle mass through strength training also helps with losing fat because metabolic rate is directly proportional to muscle mass: The more muscle mass, the higher the metabolic rate. A high metabolic rate means that a nutritionally sound diet will not lead to an increase in body fat.

Improved Performance of Physical Activities

A person with a moderate-to-high level of muscular strength and endurance can perform everyday tasks such as climbing stairs and carrying books or groceries with ease. Muscular strength and endurance are also important in recreational activities; people with poor muscle strength tire more easily and are less effective in activities like hiking, skiing, and playing tennis. Increased strength can enhance your enjoyment of recreational sports by making it possible to achieve high levels of performance and to handle advanced techniques.

Improved Muscle and Bone Health with Aging

Research has shown that good muscle strength helps people live healthier lives. A lifelong program of regular strength training prevents muscle and nerve degeneration that can compromise the quality of life and increase the risk of hip fractures and other potentially life-threatening injuries. After age thirty, people begin to lose muscle mass. As a person ages, motor nerves can become disconnected from the portion of muscle they control. Muscle physiologists estimate that by age seventy, 15 percent of the motor nerves in most people are no longer connected to muscle tissue. Aging and inactivity also cause muscles to become slower and therefore less able to perform quick, powerful movements. Strength training helps maintain motor-nerve connections and the quickness of muscles.

Osteoporosis is common in people over age fifty-five, particularly postmenopausal women. Osteoporosis leads to fractures that can be life threatening. Hormonal changes from aging account for much of the bone loss that occurs, but lack of bone stress due to inactivity and a poor diet are contributory factors. Recent research indicates that strength training can lessen bone loss even if it is taken up later in life. Increased muscle strength can also help prevent falls, which are a major cause of injury in people with osteoporosis.

What is Muscular Strength and Endurance?

Muscular strength and muscular endurance are distinct but related components of fitness. Muscular strength, the maximum amount of force a muscle can produce in a single effort, is usually assessed by measuring the maximum amount of weight a person can lift one time. This single maximal movement is referred to as one repetition maximum (1 RM).

Muscular endurance is the ability of a muscle to exert a submaximal force repeatedly or continuously overtime. This ability depends on muscular strength because a certain amount of strength is required for any muscle movement. Muscular endurance is usually assessed by counting the maximum number of repetitions of a muscular contraction a person can do. You can test the muscular endurance of a major muscle group in your body by taking the sixty-second-sit-up test or the curl-up test and the push-up test.

How Does Weight Training Work?

Muscles move the body and enable it to exert force because they move the skeleton. When a muscle contracts (shortens), it moves a bone by pulling on the tendon that attaches the muscle to the bone. Muscles consist of individual muscle cells, or muscle fibers, connected in bundles. A single muscle is made up of many bundles of muscle fibers and is covered by layers of connective tissue that hold the fibers together. Muscle fibers, in turn, are made up of smaller units called myofibrils. (When your muscles are given the signal to contract, protein filaments within the myofibrils slide across one another, causing the muscle fiber to shorten.) Weight training causes the size of individual muscle fibers to increase by increasing the number of myofibrils. Larger muscle fibers mean a larger and stronger muscle. The development of larger muscle fibers is called hypertrophy.

Muscle fibers are classified as fast-twitch or slow-twitch fibers according to their strength, speed of contraction, and energy source. Slow-twitch fibers are relatively fatigue resistant, but they don't contract as rapidly or strongly as fast-twitch fibers. The main energy system that fuels slow-twitch fibers is aerobic. Fast-twitch fibers contract more rapidly and forcefully than slow-twitch fibers but fatigue more quickly. Although oxygen is important in the energy system that fuels fast-twitch fibers, they rely more on anaerobic metabolism than slow-twitch fibers do.

Most muscles contain a mixture of slow-twitch and fast-twitch fibers. The type of fiber that acts depends on the type of work required. Endurance activities like jogging tend to use slow-twitch fibers, whereas strength and power activities like sprinting use fast-twitch fibers. Weight training can increase the size and strength of both fast-twitch and slow-twitch fibers, although fast-twitch fibers are mostly increased.

Types of Weight Training Exercises

Weight training exercises are generally classified as isometric or isotonic. Each involves a different way of using and strengthening muscles.

Isometric exercise, also called static exercise, involves applying force without movement. To perform an isometric exercise, a person can use an immovable object like a wall to provide resistance, or the individual can just tighten a muscle while remaining still (for example, tightening the abdominal muscles while sitting at a desk). In isometrics, the muscle contracts, but there is no movement.

Isometric exercises aren't as widely used as isotonic exercises because they don't develop strength throughout a joint's entire range of motion.

Isotonic (or dynamic) exercise involves applying force with movement. Isotonic exercises are the most popular type of exercises for increasing muscle strength and seem to be the most valuable for developing strength that can be transferred to other forms of physical activity. They can be performed with weight machines, free weights, or a person's own body weight (as in sit-ups or push-ups).

There are two kinds of isotonic muscle contractions: concentric and eccentric. A concentric muscle contraction occurs when the muscle applies force as it shortens. An eccentric muscle contraction occurs when the muscle applies force as it lengthens. For example, in an arm curl, the biceps muscle works concentrically as the weight is raised toward the shoulder and eccentrically as the weight is lowered.

Exercises

A complete weight training program works all the major muscle groups. It usually takes about eight to ten different exercises to get a complete workout. For overall fitness, you need to include exercises for your neck, upper back, shoulders, arms, chest, abdomen, lower back, thighs, buttocks, and calves.

The order of exercises can also be important. Do exercises for large muscle groups, or for more than one joint, before you do exercises that use small muscle groups or single joint. This allows for more effective overload of the larger, more powerful muscle groups. Small-muscle groups fatigue more easily than larger ones, and small-muscle fatigue limits your capacity to overload larger muscle groups. For example, lateral raises, which work the shoulder muscles, should be performed after bench presses, which work the chest and arms in addition to the shoulders. If you fatigue your shoulder muscles by doing lateral raises first, you won't be able to lift as much weight and effectively fatigue all the key muscle groups used during the bench press.

Resistance

The amount of weight (resistance) you lift in weight training exercises is equivalent in intensity to cardiorespiratory endurance training. It determines the way your body will adapt to weight training and how quickly these adaptations will occur. Choose weights based on your current level of muscular fitness and your fitness goals. To build strength rapidly, you should lift weights as heavy as 80 percent of your maximum capacity (1 RM). If you are more interested in building endurance, choose a lighter weight, perhaps 40-60 percent of 1 RM. For example, if your maximum capacity for the leg press is 160 pounds, you might lift 130 pounds to build strength and 80 pounds to build endurance. For a general fitness program to develop both strength and endurance, choose a weight in the middle of this range, perhaps 70 percent of 1 RM.

Because it can be time-consuming to continually reassess your maximum capacity for each exercise, you might find it easier to choose a weight based on the number of repetitions of an exercise you can perform with a given resistance. For example, find a weight that will allow your muscles to fatigue between eight and twelve repetitions.

Repetitions and Sets

In order to improve fitness, you must do enough repetitions of each exercise to fatigue your muscles. The number of repetitions needed to cause fatigue depends on the amount of resistance: The heavier the weight, the fewer repetitions to reach fatigue. In general, a heavyweight and a low number of repetitions (one to five) build strength, whereas a lightweight and a high number of repetitions (fifteen to twenty) build endurance. For a general fitness program to build both strength and endurance, try to do about eight to twelve repetitions of each exercise; a few exercises, such as abdominal crunches and calf raises, may require more. Choose a weight heavy enough to fatigue your muscles but light enough for you to complete the repetitions with good form. Due to an increased risk of injury, it is recommended that older and more frail people (approximately fifty to sixty years of age and above) perform more repetitions (ten to fifteen) using a lighter weight.

In weight training, a "set" refers to a group of repetitions of an exercise followed by a rest period. Surprisingly, exercise scientists have not identified the optimal number of sets for increasing strength. For developing strength and endurance for general fitness, a single set of each exercise is sufficient, provided you use enough resistance to fatigue your muscles. (You should just barely be able to complete the eight-to-twelve repetitions for each exercise.) Doing more than one set of each exercise may increase strength development, and most serious weight trainers do at least three sets of each exercise.

If you perform more than one set of an exercise, you need to rest long enough between sets to allow your muscles to work at a high-enough intensity to increase fitness. The length of the rest interval depends on the amount of resistance. In a program to develop a combination of strength and endurance for wellness, a rest period of one to three minutes between sets is appropriate. If you are lifting heavier loads to build maximum strength, rest three to five minutes between sets. You can save time in your workouts if you alternate sets of different exercises. Each muscle group can rest between sets while you work on other muscles.

Warm-up and Cooldown

As with cardiorespiratory endurance exercise, you should warm up before every weight training session and cool down afterward. You should do both a general warm-up—several minutes of walking or easy jogging—and a warm-up for the weight training exercises you plan to perform. For example, if you plan to do one or more sets of ten repetitions of bench presses with 125 pounds, you might do one set of ten repetitions with 50 pounds as a warm-up. Do similar warm-up exercises for each exercise in your program.

To cool down after weight training, relax for five to ten minutes after your workout. Including a period of postexercise stretching may help prevent muscle soreness. Warmed-up muscles and joints make this a particularly good time to work on flexibility.

Frequency of Exercise

For general fitness, the American College of Sports Medicine recommends a frequency of two to three days per week for weight training. Allow your muscles at least one day of rest between workouts. If you train too often, your muscles won't be able to work at a high-enough intensity to improve their fitness, and soreness and injury are more likely to result. If you enjoy weight training and would like to train more often, try working different muscle groups on alternate days. For example, work your arms and upper body one day, work your lower body the next day, and then return to upper body exercises on the third day.

A Sample Weight Training Program for General Fitness

Guidelines

Type of activity: 8-10 weight training exercises that focus on major muscle groups

Frequency: 2-3 days per week

Resistance: Weights heavy enough to cause muscle fatigue when performed for the selected number of repetitions

Repetitions: 8-12 of each exercise (10-15 with a lower weight for people over age 50-60)

Sets: 1-3 (Doing more than one set per exercise may result in faster and greater strength gains.)

SAMPLE PROGRAM				
	Exercise	Resistance (10)	Repetitions	Sets
1	Bench Press	60	10	1-3
2	Overhead Press	40	10	1-3
3	Lat Pulls	40	10	1-3
4	Lateral Raises	10	10	1-3
5	Biceps Curls	25	10	1-3
6	Squats	30	10	1-3
7	Toe Raises	25	15	1-3
8	Abdominal Curls	—	30	1-3
9	Spine Extensions	—	10	1-3
10	Neck Flexion	—	10	1-3

The Weight Training Exercises

Exercise 1—Bench Press

Muscles Developed: Pectoralis major, triceps, deltoids

Instructions:

A. Lying on a bench on your back, with your feet on the floor, grasp the bar with palms upward and hands shoulder-width apart.

B. Lower the bar to your chest. Then return it to the starting position. The bar should follow an elliptical path, during which the weight moves from a low point at the chest to a high point over the chin. If your back arches too much, try doing this exercise with your feet on the bench.

Exercise 2—Overhead Press

Muscles Developed: Deltoids, triceps, trapezius

Instructions:

This exercise can be done standing or sitting with dumbbells or barbells. The shoulder press begins with the weight at your chest.

A.   Grasp the weight with your palms facing away from you.

B.   Push the weight overhead until your arms are extended (do not lock your elbows). Then return to the starting position (weight at chest). Be careful not to arch your back excessively.

Exercise 3—Lat Pulls

Muscles Developed: Latisimus dorsi, biceps

Instructions:

Begin in a seated or kneeling position, depending on the type of lat machine and the manufacturer's instructions.

A.   Grasp the bar of the machine with arms fully extended.

B.   Slowly pull the weight down until it reaches the back of your neck. Slowly return to the starting position.

Exercise 4—Lateral Raise

Muscles Developed: Deltoids

Instructions:

A.   Stand with feet shoulder-width apart and a dumbbell in each hand. Hold the dumbbells parallel to each other.

B.   With elbows slightly bent, slowly lift both weights until they reach shoulder level. Keep your wrists in a neutral position, in-line with your forearms. Return to the starting position.

Exercise 5—Biceps Curl

Muscles Developed: Biceps, brachialis

Instructions:

A. From a standing position, grasp the bar with your palms upward and your hands shoulder-width apart.

B. Keeping your upper body rigid, flex (bend) your elbows until the bar reaches a level slightly below the collarbone. Return the bar to the starting position.

Exercise 6—Squat

Muscles Developed: Quadriceps, gluteus maximus, hamstrings, gastrocnemius

Instructions:

Stand with feet shoulder-width apart and toes pointed slightly outward.

A.   Rest the bar on the back of your shoulders, holding it there with hands facing forward.

B.   Keeping your head up and lower back straight, squat down until your thighs are almost parallel with the floor. Drive upward toward the starting position, keeping your back in a fixed position throughout the exercise.

Exercise 7—Toe Raise

Muscles Developed: Gastrocnemius, soleus

Instructions:

Stand with feet shoulder-width apart and toes pointed straight ahead.

A.   Rest the bar on the back of your shoulders, holding it there with hands facing forward.

B.   Press down with your toes while lifting your heels. Return to the starting position.

Exercise 8—Abdominal Curl

Muscles Developed: Rectus abdominis, obliques

Instructions:

A. Lie on your back on the floor with your arms folded across your chest and your feet on the floor or a bench.

B. Curl your trunk up and forward by raising your head and shoulders from the ground. Lower to the starting position.

Exercise 9—Spine Extensions

Muscles Developed: Erector spinae, gluteus maximus, hamstrings, deltoids

Instructions:

Begin on all fours with your knees below your hips and your hands below your shoulders.

Unilateral Spine Extension:

A.   Extend your right leg to the rear, and reach forward with your right arm. Keep your neck neutral and your raised arm and leg in-line with your torso. Don't arch your back or let your hip or shoulder sag. Hold this position for ten to thirty seconds. Repeat with your left leg and left arm.

Bilateral Spine Extension:

B.   Extend your left leg to the rear and reach forward with your right arm. Keep your neck neutral and your raised leg in-line with your torso. Don't arch your back or let your hip or shoulder sag. Hold this position for ten to thirty seconds. Repeat with your right leg and right arm.

Exercise 10—Neck Flexion and Lateral Flexion

Muscles Developed: Sternocleidomastoids, scaleni

Instructions:

Neck Flexion:

A. Place your hand on your forehead with fingertips pointed up. Using the muscles at the back of your neck, press your head forward and resist the pressure with the palm of your hand.

Lateral Flexion:

B. Place your hand on the right side of your face, fingertips pointed up. Using the muscles on the left side of your neck, press your head to the right and resist the pressure with the palm of your hand. Repeat on the left side.

Alternate Your Weight Training Days

If you find that you really enjoy weight training and would like to do it more than two to three days a week, alternate your workouts between upper body one day and lower body the next.

The following are exercises you will do on the day for your upper body workout:

Warm-Up

As always, begin with a five-minute aerobic warm-up to get your heart pumping and to get freshly oxygenated blood to your muscles. You can do this by marching in place, doing side steps, jogging in place, or a combination of all three.

A Few Simple Stretches

Deep Breath

1. Take a deep breath.

2. Inhale through the nose as your arms flow out to the sides and up overhead. Exhale out the mouth as your arms slowly come down to your sides.

3. Repeat three times.

Full-Body Stretch

This is a great stretch for your whole body, especially your arms, shoulders, and spine. You can do this one either sitting or standing.

1. Lift your arms above your head and reach as high as you can.

2. Make sure you breathe while holding this stretch for five to fifteen seconds.

3. Bring your arms down in front of you and relax.

Modification:

Side Stretch—Slowly bend slightly to the left and then to the right.

Triceps Stretch

Designed to stretch the muscles of the backs of your upper arms, it can be performed either sitting or standing. In addition to doing this one at the beginning and the end of your workout, you might find it beneficial to perform the stretch in between exercises.

1. Raise your right arm above you and bend the elbow so your right hand is behind your neck.

2. With your left hand, grasp your right elbow and gently pull the elbow behind your head.

3. Hold the stretch for fifteen to twenty seconds.

4. You should feel a nice stretch in your right triceps.

5. Relax and repeat the stretch on the left arm.

Your Upper Body Workout

Pec Press (with weights)

Muscles Worked: Chest (pectoralis)

Instructions:

1. Lie on your back with your knees bent and your feet on the floor.

2. With the weights in your hands, slowly bend your arms so that your elbows are parallel to your shoulders.

3. Push the weights straight up so that your arms are extended directly over your chest.

4. Return to starting position.

5. Repeat the movement.

Do three sets of eight-to-twelve reps each. Rest fifteen seconds between sets.

Chest Flys (with weights)

Muscles Worked: Chest (pectoralis)

Instructions:

1. Lie on your back on the floor with your knees bent and your feet flat on the floor.

2. Hold the weights in your hands with your arms extended straight-out at shoulder level, above your chest, with palms facing inward.

3. Slowly lower your arms to your side, keeping them bent at the same angle throughout the movement.

4. Slowly return your arms to the starting position by squeezing your chest as if you're making a cleavage and repeating the movement.

Do three sets of eight-to-twelve reps each. Rest fifteen seconds between sets.

Biceps Curl (with weights)

Muscles Worked: Biceps

Instructions:

1. Sit on the floor with your legs crossed in front of you. Your back should be straight and your abs tight.

2. With an underhand grip, hold the weights at your sides with your arms extended.

3. Exhale as you slowly raise the weights toward your upper arms and shoulders, bending your elbows.

4. Hold momentarily and return your hands to the starting position. Be sure that you keep your elbows close to your body throughout the movement.

Do three sets of eight-to-twelve reps each. Rest fifteen seconds between sets.

Lateral-Side Raises (with weights)

Muscles Worked: Shoulders (deltoids)

Instructions:

1. Stand with your feet shoulder-width apart, abs tight, back straight, and knees slightly bent.

2. Hold weights at your side.

3. Raise the weights out to your sides. Arms should be straight and palms down. Return to the starting position.

4. Continue to complete lateral-side raises up and down.

Do three sets of eight-to-twelve reps each. Rest fifteen seconds between sets.

Triceps Toner (with weights)

Muscles Worked: Back of arms (triceps)

Instructions:

1. Stand with your feet shoulder-width apart and knees slightly bent with weights in your hands. Keep your abs tight, back flat, and bend slightly forward at the waist.

2. Raise your elbows so that the upper part of your arms is parallel with the floor. Keep your elbows close to your body.

3. Straighten your arms. Be sure to squeeze your triceps as you do so.

4. Return your hands to the starting position, pause, and repeat the movement.

Do three sets of eight-to-twelve reps each. Rest fifteen seconds between sets.

The Chest Press

Muscles Worked: Chest and back of upper arms (pecs and triceps)

Instructions:

1. Lie with your back flat on a bench and with your knees bent. Keep your back flat against the bench with little or no arch. Hold the appropriate weight in each hand, slightly above chest level and with your palms facing forward.

2. Contract your abdominal muscles. Gradually raise both dumbbells up until your arms are fully extended above your chest. Do not lock your elbows. Slowly return the dumbbells back to the starting position. Control your movements throughout the entire exercise, exhaling when raising the dumbbells and inhaling on the return.

3. Keep your head and back firmly against the bench throughout the entire exercise.

Do three sets of eight-to-twelve reps each. Rest fifteen seconds between sets.

The Shoulder Press

Muscles Worked: Shoulders

Instructions:

1. Sit upright in a chair with your back supported and your feet flat on the floor. Keep your back flat against the back of the chair with little or no arch. Hold the appropriate weight in each hand, slightly above shoulder level and with your palms facing forward. Keep your elbows out to the side.

2. Contract your abdominal muscles. Keeping your palms facing forward, raise the weights up and inward until the inside ends of the dumbbells are nearly touching each other and are directly overhead. Do not lock your elbows. Pause, then lower the dumbbells slowly to the starting position. Control your movements throughout the entire exercise, exhaling upon raising the dumbbells and inhaling on the return.

Do three sets of eight-to-twelve reps each. Rest fifteen seconds between sets.

The Triceps Extension

Muscles Worked: Back of upper arms (triceps)

Instructions:

1. Stand straight with your feet slightly apart and your knees slightly bent. Using an interlocking grip, hold a dumbbell of the appropriate weight above your head with your arms fully extended.

2. Contract your abdominal muscles. Slowly lower the dumbbell back behind your head and neck while keeping your elbows in place above your head. Continue until your forearms are parallel to the floor.

3. Control your movements and maintain your posture throughout the entire exercise. Pause, then gradually raise the dumbbell back up to the starting position. Inhale while lowering the dumbbell down and exhale when raising it up.

Do three sets of eight-to-twelve reps each. Rest fifteen seconds between sets.

One-Arm Row (with weights)

Muscles Worked: Upper back (latisimus dorsi, rhomboid),
back of shoulders (posterior deltoid)

Instructions:

1. Stand with your feet apart, left foot in front of the right.

2. Bend your knees slightly, and keep your abs tight.

3. Rest the palm of your left hand on your left thigh. Holding the weight in your right hand, let your arm extend to the floor.

4. Pull the weight up to your armpit, then lower it back to the starting position and repeat.

Do three sets of eight-to-twelve reps each. Rest fifteen seconds between sets.

Push-Ups

Muscles Worked: Chest (pectoralis), shoulders (anterior deltoid), triceps

Instructions:

1. Kneel on the floor with your ankles crossed and your hands out in front of you on the floor.

2. Straighten your back, with abs tight and your head in a natural position.

3. Slowly bend your elbows, and lower your chest to the floor.

4. Straighten your elbows, and return to the starting position.

Do three sets of eight-to-twelve reps each. Rest fifteen seconds between sets.

Your Lower Body Workouts and Exercises

Warm-Up

As always, begin with a five-minute aerobic warm-up to get your heart pumping and to get freshly oxygenated blood to your muscles. You can do this by marching in place, doing side steps, jogging in place, or a combination of all three.

Next—A Few Simple Stretches

Quad Stretch

Your quadriceps is the four muscles in the front of your thighs. They are among the largest and strongest muscle groups in your body and are used in every activity.

1.   Lie on your side with your legs together.

2.   Bend your right leg behind you, and grasp the foot or the ankle.

3.   Gently pull your foot toward your buttocks.

4.   When you feel tension in the front of your thighs, hold the stretch fifteen to twenty seconds.

5.   Switch sides and repeat the movement with the left leg.

Reach for Toes

This is a great stretch for the backs of your legs (hamstrings) and your lower back (erector spinae). Placing the towel under your buttocks will assist you in achieving proper form, making the exercise easier and more effective. The correct technique is to keep your back straight and to lengthen the space between your sternum and pelvic bone. Don't hunch shoulders forward.

1. Sit on the floor, place a towel under your buttocks, and keep your legs straight-out in front of you.

2. Sit up with your back straight, abs tight, and toes pointing to the ceiling.

3. Exhale as you bend forward, reaching your hands toward your toes.

4. Be sure that you keep your legs and back as straight as you possibly can.

5. Hold the stretch for fifteen to twenty seconds, relax, and repeat.

Hamstring Stretch

This is a wonderful stretch for the back of the legs (hamstrings). It is especially useful if your lower back is bothering you. As with the rest of your stretches, be sure to breathe, relax, and never bounce.

1. Lie on your back on the floor with your knees bent and your feet on the floor.

2. Raise your right leg up, and pull it toward your chest. You can use a towel to assist you.

3. Hold the stretch for fifteen to twenty seconds.

4. Lower the leg and repeat the stretch with the left leg.

Lower Body Exercises

Basic Stomach Crunch

Muscles Worked: Abdominals (rectus abdominis)

Instructions:

1. Lie on your back with your knees bent and your feet on the floor. (If you are a beginner, or have neck problems, use a pillow under your neck and head.)

2. Press your lower back firmly into the floor. There should be no arch in your back at all.

3. Rest your head in your hands, but keep your neck and shoulders relaxed.

4. Tighten your abdominals and slowly lift your shoulders up off the floor (about six inches).

5. Exhale as you crunch. Keep your elbows back and chin up as if you have an apple between your chin and chest.

6. Slowly lower your shoulders back to the floor and repeat.

Do three sets of eight-to-twelve crunches each. Rest fifteen seconds between sets.

Basic Squats

Muscles Worked: Thighs (quadriceps), buttocks (gluteals), hamstrings

Instructions:

1. Stand with your feet a little wider than your hips. Your back should be straight and your abs tight.

2. Place your hands on your hips.

3. Bend your knees and begin to squat. Feel as though you're sitting back, with your body weight through your heels. Hips should move behind your heels, like you are lowering yourself into a chair. Simultaneously raise your hands in front of you—this will help you balance.

4. As you stand back up, exhale and squeeze your buttocks. Repeat.

5. Never go lower than a ninety-degree angle.

Do three sets of eight-to-twelve crunches each. Rest fifteen seconds between sets.

Basic Outer Thigh Leg Lift

Muscles Worked: Outer thigh (abductors)

Instructions:

1. Lie on the floor with your left side down. Your head, shoulders, and hips should all be aligned.

2. Bend your left leg, putting your right hand down in front of you for balance.

3. Keeping your right leg straight and your foot flexed, slowly raise your leg. Lower it back to the floor, then repeat. This is a very short movement, so be careful not to raise your leg too high. You should be focusing on the outer thigh of your top leg.

Do three sets of eight-to-twelve leg lifts on each leg.

Basic Inner Thigh Lift

Muscles Worked: Inner thigh (adductors)

Instructions:

1. Lie on the floor on your left side. Your head, shoulders, and hips should all be aligned.

2. Bend your right leg and place it on the floor in front of you.

3. Slowly raise your left leg off the floor to a comfortable height. Try to keep it straight.

4. Pause at the top of the movement, then lower the leg back to the floor. Repeat.

5. Your left foot should remain flexed and parallel to the floor throughout the movement.

Do three sets of eight-to-twelve leg lifts on each leg.

Walking Lunges

Muscles Worked: Thighs (quadriceps), buttocks (gluteals), hamstrings

Instructions:

1. Hold weights at your sides (weights optional). Start with your feet about shoulder-width apart.

2. Take a step with one foot. As you take your step, bend your back knee toward the floor. Be sure you don't bang your knee on the floor. Your body weight should be on your front heel and on your back toes.

3. Rise back up, and as you do, bring your back foot forward to return to the starting position.

4. Take giant steps forward, alternating legs.

Do three sets of eight-to-twelve lunges each. Rest fifteen seconds between sets.

Calf Raises

Muscles Worked: Calves (gastrocnemius)

Instructions:

1. Stand with your feet together. Place your hands on the back of a chair for balance.

2. Raise up on your toes so that you are on the balls of your feet. As you rise, be sure to really squeeze your calves.

3. Lower your heels back to the floor and repeat. This exercise can also be done one leg at a time to make it a little tougher.

Do three sets of eight-to-twelve leg raises. Rest fifteen seconds between sets.

Oblique Crunch

Muscles Worked: Obliques

Instructions:

1. Lie on your back with knees bent and feet flat on the floor. Make sure the small of the back is pressed into the floor.

2. Contract the abdominals as you lift your head and shoulders about six inches from the floor.

3. Twist slightly to the side, reaching your hands to the outside of your right thigh. Hold the reach, and try to keep shoulders off the floor, pulsing (lifting up and down). Those of you who need support for your neck, place your hands behind your head. Your abdominal muscles should be contracted the entire time. Your goal is to keep the shoulder blades off the floor.

4. Hold the reach while pulsing. After completing three sets on the right side, repeat on the left side.

Do three sets of eight-to-twelve crunches each.

Upper Body Firmer (with weights)

Muscles Worked: Shoulders (posterior deltoid), upper back (rhomboids)

Instructions:

1. Sit in a chair. Lean forward so your chest is near your thighs.

2. With weights in your hands, slowly lift your arms straight-out to the sides, your pinkies up.

3. Squeeze your shoulder blades together. Return to the starting position and repeat the movement. Make sure that your movement is slow and deliberate; try not to swing the weights.

Do three sets of eight to twelve each.

Buttocks Firmer

Muscles Worked: Buttocks (gluteals)

Instructions:

1. Kneel on the floor with your elbows and hands on the floor.

2. Be sure to keep your back flat, abs tight, and your hips square to the floor.

3. Raise your right leg from the floor, keeping it bent at a right angle. Your upper leg and right foot should be parallel to the floor.

4. Slowly raise your knee up and down, pressing your foot toward the ceiling, squeezing your buttocks.

Do three sets of eight-to-twelve reps for each leg. Rest fifteen seconds between sets.

Power Lunge

Muscles Worked: Thighs (quadriceps), hamstrings, buttocks (gluteals)

Instructions:

1. Start with your feet about shoulder-width apart (weights optional).

2. Take a step forward with one foot. Make sure front knee stays at a ninety-degree angle. Keep your knee in a line with your ankle.

3. As you step forward, bend your back knee. Be sure you don't bang it on the floor. Your weight should be balanced between your back toes and your front heel.

4. Push back to the starting position bringing legs together, and repeat alternating your legs.

Do three sets of eight-to-twelve reps each. Rest fifteen seconds between sets.

Flexibility

Flexibility

Flexibility is the ability of a joint to move through its full range of motion—it's extremely important for general fitness and wellness. The smooth and easy performance of everyday and recreational activities is impossible if flexibility is poor.

Flexibility is a highly adaptable physical fitness component. It increases in response to a regular program of stretching exercises and decreases with inactivity. Flexibility is also specific; good flexibility in one joint does not necessarily mean good flexibility in another. Flexibility can be increased through stretching exercises for all major joints.

There are two basic types of flexibility: static and dynamic. Static flexibility refers to the ability to assume and maintain an extended position at one end or point in a joint's range of motion; it is what most people mean by the term "flexibility." Dynamic flexibility, unlike static flexibility, involves movement. It is the ability to move a joint quickly through its range of motion with little resistance.

Static flexibility depends on many factors, including the structure of a joint and the tightness of muscles, tendons, and ligaments that are attached to it. Dynamic flexibility is dependent on static flexibility; but it also involves such factors as strength, coordination, and resistance to movement. Dynamic flexibility can be important for both daily activities and sports. However, because static flexibility is easier to measure and better researched, most assessment tests and stretching programs target static flexibility.

Benefits of Flexibility and Stretching Exercises

Good flexibility provides benefits for the entire muscular and skeletal system; it may also prevent injuries and soreness and improve performance in sports and other activities.

Joint Health

Good flexibility is essential to good joint health. When the muscles and other tissues that support a joint are tight, the joint is subject to abnormal stresses that can cause joint deterioration. For example, tight thigh muscles cause excessive pressure on the kneecap, leading to pain in the knee joint. Tight shoulder muscles can compress sensitive soft tissues in the shoulder, leading to pain and disability in the joint. Poor joint flexibility can also cause abnormalities in joint lubrication, leading to deterioration of the sensitive cartilage cells lining the joint. Pain and further joint injury can result.

Improved flexibility can greatly improve your quality of life, particularly as you get older. Aging decreases the natural elasticity of muscles, tendons, and joints, resulting in stiffness. The problem is compounded if you have arthritis. Flexibility exercises improve the elasticity in your tissues, making it easier to move your body. When you're flexible, every activity becomes easier.

Reduction of Postexercise Muscle Soreness

Delayed onset muscle soreness occurring one to two days after exercise is thought to be caused by damage to the muscle fibers and supporting connective tissue. Some studies have shown that stretching after exercise decreases the degree of muscle soreness.

Relief of Aches and Pains

Flexibility exercises help relieve pain that develops from stress or prolonged sitting. Studying or working in one place for a long time can cause your muscles to become tense. Stretching helps relieve tension, so you can go back to work refreshed and effective.

Improved Body Position and Strength

Good flexibility lets a person assume more efficient body positions and exert force through a greater range of motion. For example, swimmers with more flexible shoulders have stronger strokes because they can pull their arms through the water in the optimal position. Flexible joints and muscles let you move more fluidly without constraint. Some studies also suggest that flexibility training enhances strength development.

Maintenance of Good Posture

Good flexibility also contributes to body symmetry and good posture. Bad postural habits can gradually change your body structures. Sitting in a slumped position, for example, can lead to tightness in the muscles in the front of your chest and overstretching and looseness in the upper spine, causing a rounding of the upper back. This condition, called kyphosis, is common in older people. It may be prevented by doing stretching exercises regularly.

Relaxation

Flexibility exercises are a great way to relax. Studies have shown that doing flexibility exercises reduces mental tension, slows your breathing rate, and reduces blood pressure.

Assessing Flexibility

Because flexibility is specific to each joint, there are no tests of general flexibility. The most commonly used flexibility test is the sit-and-reach test. This test rates the flexibility of the muscles in the lower back and hamstrings. Flexibility in these muscles may be important in preventing low-back pain.

Sit-and-Reach Test

Equipment: A flexibility box or measuring device. If you make your own measuring device, use two pieces of wood twelve inches high, attached at right angles to each other. Use a ruler or yardstick to measure the extent of reach. With the low numbers of the ruler toward the person being tested, set the six-inch mark of the ruler at the foot line of the box.

Preparation: Warm up your muscles with some low-intensity activity such as marching or jogging in place for five minutes.

Instructions:

1. Remove your shoes, and sit facing the flexibility box with your knees fully extended and your feet about four inches apart. Your feet should be flat against the box.

2. Reach as far forward as you can with palms down and one hand placed on top of the other. Hold the position of maximum reach for one to two seconds. Keep your knees locked at all times.

3. Repeat the stretch two times. Your score is the most distant point reached with the fingertips of both hands on the third trial, measured to the nearest quarter of an inch.

Rating Your Flexibility

Find your score in the table below to determine your flexibility rating.

Ratings for Sit-and-Reach Test (Men)				
Age	Very Poor	Poor	Moderate	High	Very High
15-19	below 5.25	5.25-6.75	7.00-8.75	9.00-10.75	above 10.75
20-29	below 5.50	5.50-7.00	7.25-8.75	9.00-11.00	above 11.00
30-39	below 4.75	4.75-6.50	6.75-8.50	8.75-10.25	above 10.25
40-49	below 2.75	2.75-5.00	5.25-6.75	7.00-10.25	above 9.25
50-59	below 2.00	2.00-5.00	5.25-6.50	6.75-9.25	above 9.25
60 and over	below 1.75	1.75-3.25	3.50-5.25	5.50-8.50	above 8.50

Ratings for Sit-and-Reach Test (Women)				
Age	Very Poor	Poor	Moderate	High	Very High
15-19	below 7.25	7.25-8.75	9.00-10.50	10.75-12.25	above 12.25
20-29	below 6.75	6.75-8.50	8.75-10.00	10.25-11.50	above 11.50
30-39	below 6.50	6.50-8.00	8.25-9.50	9.75-11.50	above 11.50
40-49	below 5.50	5.50-7.25	7.50-8.75	9.00-10.50	above 10.50
50-59	below 5.50	5.50-7.25	7.50-8.50	8.75-10.75	above 10.75
60 and over	below 4.75	4.75-6.00	6.25-7.75	8.00-9.25	above 9.25

Intensity and Duration of Flexibility Exercises

For each exercise, slowly apply stretch to your muscles to the point of slight tension or mild discomfort. Hold the stretch for ten to thirty seconds. As you hold the stretch, the feeling of slight tension should slowly subside. At that point, try to stretch a bit farther. Throughout the stretch, try to relax and breathe easily. Rest for about thirty to sixty seconds between each stretch, and do at least four repetitions of each stretch.

Frequency of Flexibility Training

The American College of Sports Medicine recommends that stretching exercises be performed a minimum of two to three days per week. Many people do flexibility training more often—three to five days per week—for even greater benefits. It's best to stretch when your muscles are warm, so try incorporating stretching into your cooldown after cardiorespiratory-endurance exercise or weight training. Stretching can also be a part of your warm-up, but it's best to increase the temperature of your muscles first by doing a five-minute warm-up of marching or jogging in place.

Flexibility Exercises

Head Turns and Tilts

Areas Stretched: Neck, upper back

Instructions:

Head Turns: Turn your head to the right and hold the stretch. Repeat to the left.

Head Tilts: Tilt your head to the left and hold the stretch. Repeat to the right.

Variation: Place your right palm on your right cheek. Try to turn your head to the right as you resist with your hand. Repeat on the left side.

The 30 minute

Express Fit Workout!

This is it! Your answer!, My answer. Have the body you want and deserve in just 30 minutes a day.

I have always loved my workouts. They destressed me, made me feel strong, and I looked pretty good. It was my little gift to myself, but when I started working the Oncology Unit at a medical center, my work days were 14 to 16 hours long. Not only did I have no time to exercise on the days that I worked, I was so tired on my day off that my usual 1 hour to hour ½ workouts were never accomplished. I just didn't have the stamina. As months went by I started to notice the definition in my muscle tone changing, not to mention the additional 5-10 lbs I put on. This was not going to work. How could I accomplish a full body workout in a short period of time? The express fit workout was born.

For maximum fitness results you need do both cardio exercise to lose weight and speed up your metabolism, and do weight training to tone and strengthen muscles. Normally these two exercises would take at least an hour, but by combining them, you can get the benefits of both in only 30 minutes.

What you will need—Hand weights
　　　　　　　—Jump rope
　　　　　　　—clock with a second hand

—We will alternate a weight training rep with a 1 minute cardio interval.

Example start by marching in place 1 minute. Immediately pick up your hand weights and do 1 set 8-12 lateral raises when done, without a break, do 1 minute of jumping rope. After 1 minute immediately pick up your hand weights and do 2nd set 8-12 lateral raises. After 2nd set immediately do 1 minute of forward lunges (you may alternate legs during the one minute) following the forward lunges immediately march in place for one full minute. Your heartrate needs to stay elevated the entire time. Try not to take breaks if you can. Keep a water bottle close by for hydration. You can substitute jumping jacks for either the marching or jump rope if you'd like. The lunges are very important because they are not only working your heart, but are conditioning your quadriceps, hamstrings, gluetes, and hip flexes. Once you have done this routine several times, it will become 2nd nature. Put on your favorite music, have fun, and in 30 minutes you have completed a challenging full body cardio/strength training workout!

Across-the-Body Stretch

Areas Stretched: Shoulders, upper back

Instructions:

Keeping your back straight, cross your left arm in front of your body and grasp it with your right hand. Stretch your arm, shoulders, and back by gently pulling your arm as close to your body as possible. Repeat the stretch with your right arm.

Variation: Bend your right arm over and behind your head. Grasp your right hand with your left, and gently pull your arm until you feel the stretch. Repeat for your left arm.

Upper-Back Stretch

Areas Stretched: Upper back

Instructions:

Stand with your feet shoulder-width apart, knees slightly bent, and pelvis tucked under. Clasp your hands in front of your body, and press your palms forward.

Variation: In the same position, wrap your arms around your body as if you were giving yourself a hug.

Lateral Stretch

Areas Stretched: Trunk muscles

Instructions:

Stand with your feet shoulder-width apart, knees slightly bent, and pelvis tucked under. Raise one arm over your head and bend sideways from the waist. Support your trunk by placing the hand or forearm of your other arm on your thigh or hip for support. Be sure you bend directly sideways and don't move your body below the waist. Repeat on the other side.

Forward Lunge

Areas Stretched: Hip, front of thigh (quadriceps)

Instructions:

Step forward and flex your forward knee, keeping your knee directly above your ankle. Stretch your other leg back so that it is parallel to the floor. Press your hips forward and down to stretch. Your arms can be at your sides, on top of your knee, or on the ground for balance. Repeat on the other side.

Side Lunge

Areas Stretched: Inner thigh, hip, calf

Instructions:

Stand in a wide straddle with your legs turned out from your hip joints and your hands on your thighs. Lunge to one side by bending one knee and keeping the other leg straight. Keep your knee directly over your ankle; do not bend it more than ninety degrees. Repeat on the other side.

Trunk Rotation

Areas Stretched: Trunk, outer thigh and hip, lower back

Instructions:

Sit with your right leg straight, left leg bent and crossed over the right knee, and left hand on the floor next to your left hip. Turn your trunk as far as possible to the left by pushing against your left leg with your right forearm or elbow. Keep your left foot on the floor. Repeat on the other side.

Alternate Leg Stretch

Areas Stretched: Back of the thigh (hamstring), hip, knee, ankle, buttocks

Instructions:

Lie flat on your back with both legs straight.

A.   Grasp your left leg behind the thigh and pull into your chest.

B.   Hold this position and then extend your left leg toward the ceiling.

C.   Hold this position, and then bring your left knee back to your chest and pull your toes toward your shin with your left hand. Stretch the back of the leg by attempting to straighten your knee.

Repeat for the other leg.

Modified Hurdler Stretch

Areas Stretched: Back of the thigh (hamstring), lower back

Instructions:

Sit with your right leg straight and your left leg tucked close to your body. Reach toward your right foot as far as possible. Repeat for the other leg.

Variation: As you stretch forward, alternately flex and point the foot of your extended leg.

Lower Leg Stretch

Areas Stretched: Back of the lower leg (calf, soleus, Achilles tendon)

Instructions:

Stand with one foot about one to two feet in front of the other, with both feet pointing forward.

A. Keeping your back leg straight, lunge forward by bending your front knee and pushing your rear heel backward. Hold this position.

B. Then pull your back foot in slightly, and bend your back knee. Shift your weight to your back leg. Hold.

Repeat on the other side.

Express Fit Workout

Warm-up march in place 3-5 minutes

1st exercise lateral raise w/weights 1 set 8-12
>   1 minute marching
>   2nd set lateral raise w/weights 1 set 8-12
>   1 minute jump rope
>   3rd set lateral raise w/weights 1 set
>   1 minute forward lunges

2nd Exercise Overhead Press
>   3 sets of 8-12 followed each time with 1 minute cardio of your choice.

3rd Exercise Biceps Curl
>   3 sets of 8-12 exercises followed each time with 1 minute cardio in between sets.

4th Exercise triceps toner
>   3 sets of 8-12 followed each time with 1 minute forward lunges

5 Upper body firmer
>   Do three sets of eight to twelve each with power lunges in between each set for one minute

6. Oblique twist
>   Take a heavy 15lb weight (you may go lighter if you need to. Stand with feet shoulder width apart hold hands on each end of the weight with it in front of your body, elbows bent right below your chest. Twist your trunk eight to 12x to the right and then 8 to 12x to the left. Repeat 3 times do one minute of cardio between each set.

Yes, you did it!

30 minutes and you did a complete full body workout with cardio!

Spiritual Fitness

Lets be real! We are all exposed to so many stresses in our lives, it is hard to keep it all straight. There is so much "white noise" going on, the voices in our own head are going a million directions all at once. The irony here is that in the big picture of it all, all those little worries really mean nothing. We spend so much time and energy worrying about this and taking care of that, we forget to just take some time to check in with ourselves and see whats really going on.

There are a few techniques you can use to help "ground" yourself during the day. They are simple and don't take alot of time. Like anything it will be a conscious effort at first, and then after a while will become second nature.

I feel that most of us feel guilty about taking time for ourselves, but the truth is if you don't take good care of you—You can't take care of anyone else.

Meditation

The Buddha reached enlightenment through meditation and devoted the rest of his life to teaching others what he had learned.

> "All you need is deep within you waiting to unfold and reveal itself. All you have to do is be still and take time to seek for what is within, and you will surely find it."
>
> Eileen Caddy.

Meditation is now being recognized for its health benefits. Clinical studies into the effects of meditation have shown reductions in migraines, insomnia, irritable bowel syndrome, premenstrual syndrome, anxiety and panic attacks, as well as lower levels of stress hormones, lower blood pressure, and improved circulation. They have also shown that meditation can help control pulse and respiratory rates. Doctors are now recommending meditation exercises and relaxation techniques to their patients. Meditation helps us restore balance. It helps us "ground" our energy to the earth and the rest of the universe. Many Eastern philosophies believe that as well as containing oxygen, air also contains vital energy (known as prana in India, Ch'i in China, and Ki in Japan). By performing conscious breathing exercises you can accumulate this energy and revitalize both your mind and your body.

It all starts with the breath.

To breath properly, you must first be aware of it. Sit in a comfortable position with your eyes open or closed. Place one hand on your chest and the other over your diaphragm just below the breast bone. Breathe in slowly through your nose, and try to breathe so that the hand on your chest remains relatively still.

Hold your breath for a few seconds, then breathe out slowly through your nose. Release as much air as possible. Repeat several times. There are several types of meditations, but they are all focused on quieting the mind. The main objective is to control the mind and live in this very moment. Do not let the mind wonder and worry about things in the past or what you are going to do in the future.

Right here right now is the only truth you know. Open all your senses to this very moment. What do you hear? What do you smell? What is your intuition telling you? This is also known as mindful meditation.

Another type or meditation is called concentrative meditation. This focuses your attention on something specific, such as the intake or breath or a specific image, or a repetative phrase.

How to Meditate

Learning to meditate takes practice like aquiring any other skill. There is no "right" way to meditate but there are a few simple things you can do to make it easier.

— a quiet place where you will not be disturbed.
— regular practice, preferably for 15 minutes a day at the same time of day
— meditation in the morning helps you feel calm and centered for the rest of the day.
— an empty stomach, the flow of the universal energy can move through your body when there are no obstructions.
— A comfortable position. Sitting with your legs crossed and hands palm faced up on your knees.
— Focus on the sound of your breath. If your mind wonders—go back to your breath.

Clearing Your Chakras

According to ancient wisdom there are seven major energy centers in each of us—our "chakras". Chakras are great centers of energy in the body. Although they are invisible to the eye, these spinning wheels of spiritual energy keep our bodies and spirits in balance.

The seven main chakras of the body are located between the base of the spine and the top of the head.

As our ancient ancestors knew and Einstein proved, each of us is made up of energy—the same invisible energy that everything else in the universe is made up of. That is what we call the Universal Energy Field.

Each of the seven chakras are associated with different parts of your being. If a certain chakra is "blocked" it can affect the area in your life it is connected to.

The first chakra is located at the base of your spine and is red in color. It is your root chakra, associated with your primal life energy location.

The second chakra, or sacral chakras, is located at the level of the lower abdomen. It is associated with sexuality, sensuality, and reproduction.

The third chakra, or solar plexus chakra, is located at the solar plexus area (this is high at the back of the abdomen, just between the ribs and navel). This wheel of energy governs inner power, the will, and self-confidence.

The fourth chakra, or heart chakra, is positioned at the level of the heart. It is associated with relationships, as well as love, compassion, and emotions in general.

The fifth chakra, or throat chakra, is located in the throat area. It is connected to expression, communication, and also with our creative impulses.

The sixth chakra, or brow chakra, is positioned at the level of the forehead, between the eyebrows. It is associated with imagination, clarity or thought, intuition, and dreams, as well as our psychic abilities.

The seventh chakra, or crown chakra, is situated on the top of the head. It governs understanding, higher consciousness, and our link with universal spirit and the devine.

To clear your chakras first sit in a comfortable position. This can be done anywhere, even while you are driving. Imagine a glowing white diamond above your head. Imagine a white light coming down out of the diamond going through the top of your head all the way down your spinal cord to your red root chakra.

Imagine that this white light is feeding vital energy into the red chakra. Then visualize the red chakra spinning with vibrant energy in a clockwise direction. Feel the energy at your base. Spend a few moments "feeding" your root chakra. When you are done imagine the white light going back up your spine, through the top of your head, back into the glowing diamond. Continue the same process but now visualize the white diamond light going down your spine and feeding your second chakra the orange sacral chakra. Picture a swirling ball of orange energy getting bigger and brighter in a clockwise direction. Stay here for a few minutes then bring the white light back up your spine to the diamond shape above your head. Continue this process until all seven chakras are swirling and open with vibrant energy.

You should connect the chakras by color.
Base chakra—red
Sacral chakra—orange
Solar Plexus chakra—yellow
Heart chakra—green
Throat chakra—sky blue
Brow chakra—indigo
Crown chakra—violet

This is a very simple practice and can be done anywhere. You will be amazed how clear you will feel.

Affirmations

The power of the mind is the strongest force there is. Everything we do has a ripple effect. If I make a decision to hurt someone, that person then reacts to the situation, maybe by getting upset with someone else, then that person goes on to carry that energy etc. etc. We have proved that our thoughts are energy. And energy cannot vanish it can only change form. Our thoughts and beliefs serve to create our reality. Because of this, changing our thoughts can change our lives. A negative thought will grow as much as a positive one and will affect our life accordingly.

Whatever we create, it starts with a thought first. The thought creates an image, a form, which magnetizes energy to flow into the image and eventually manifest itself on the physical plane. We will create, and therefore attract into our lives the beliefs and desires that we focus on the most intensely.

Positive affirmations need a conscious effort to perfect. Everytime your mind says something in the negative tense, rephrase the same thought in a positive statement. For example, if you are on your way to interview for a new job, and inside your head you hear "I'll never get this job". Stop yourself right there and say "I will get this job." Go even further by stating examples of why you will get this job. Say them aloud. Say them with conviction.

Practice affirmations everyday. I particularly love doing them in the car on my way to work in the morning. Say aloud all the wonderful things that you are. Picture where you would like to be in 5 years and then see yourself there. See everything about it. Affirm it aloud and let the energy magnetize it to you! Enjoy!

Alpha vs Beta

Scientists have said that we only use 10% of our brains. What is going on in the other 90%?

We are connected to all things through electrical waves. Depending on what time of day it is, how stressed we are, what we have injested, we are either emitting alpha waves or beta waves.

The left side of the brain deals with thinking, speaking, and writing. When we are fully awake and in a busy, thinking state of mind, the brain emits faster electrical patterns called "beta" waves. In this state we are able to rationalize and think about the past and future.

The right side of the brain deals with intuition, imagination, and feeling. When we are sensing something—and we are in a receptive rather than an active state, the brain emits slower electrical patterns called "alpha" waves. In the alpha state we are more passive and open to our feelings. The alpha state is most likely to happen when we live in the present rather than in the future or the past. It often happens just before or after sleep (but not during sleep—when we are sleeping the brain emits other waves, called theta and delta). When we are awake we are usually in beta most of the time. Meditation helps to restore the balance by increasing our time spent in alpha: it helps us to recover feeling and to experience the world directly, in the present, before the sensations become "interpreted" by the left side of the brain.

Spiritual fitness tip—feed and nurture your spirit. We are here on earth to be challenged and have all types of experiences to help us grow spiritually. Embrace every opportunity. Even a situation that causes pain and suffering is a little gift. Keep in mind that pain is temporary, at the end a greater understanding on a higher level will be achieved. (If you are open to it).

Spiritual fitness tip—Always listen to your gut instincts. Stand in your truth of what you feel inside. It is always right, even if at the time it does not seem logical. Trust it!

Love and Peace,
Suzanne

Transpersonal Counseling

The definition of transpersonal is beyond the personal. It encompasses the mind, body, and spirit.

When a transpersonal counseling session takes place, it is started with a quiet meditative state in order to silence the mind and call forth a persons higher self.

We believe that there are no "mistakes" in life, only lessons that we have asked to be given in order to learn from them and have a better understanding of the meaning of life. It is our belief that before we came into our physical body, we actually agreed with God, the path and circumstances we would experience in this lifetime. We have guides and angels that are assigned to us and actually stay with us and help us every step of way. It is through transpersonal counseling that we connect with our higher power and see the whole picture of what we are experiencing here on earth and what we are suppose to learn from it.

It is important to remember that we are all connected. Every person, every living thing, we are ultimately one. There is no one higher or lower, better, or worse. when something happens in life that is particularly challenging – and of course they happen, have faith. What may seem like a terrible experience will reveal its "gift" at some point and it will all make sense. The ultimate goal is love and forgiveness, it is also the ultimate reward.

Reiki

There is a life force energy that connects all things to one another. It goes beyond centuries and across all cultures. It is called different names in different languages, but it is the same vibrant life force.

Reiki is the technique that is used to allow the "life force" to flow through the practitioner and given to the person receiving the healing. The existence of reiki energy has been verified by several scientific experiments, and major medical centers now offer reiki as part of their holistic healing services to their patients.

Reiki promotes healing by guiding an unlimited supply of "life energy" into a patient. A treatment feels like a wonderful glowing radiance that flows through you and surrounds you. It creates many beneficial effects including relaxation and feelings of peace, security and well being. Experience one for yourself.

Your Thirty-Day Fitness Program

At this point, you have gathered all the information on healthy eating, exercise, and how both contribute to preventing disease. Now it's time to take action.

If losing weight is one of your goals (and it is for most of us), you need to create a negative caloric balance. Taking off pounds is a mathematical equation. You must take in lesser calories than you burn off in a given day. One pound is equal to 3,500 calories. Losing weight properly should be consistent at about one to two pounds per week. I suggest that your goal be one pound a week.

Complete the following calculations to determine your weekly and daily negative caloric balance goals and the number of weeks to achieve your target weight.

Current weight: _____ lb.
Minus target weight: _____ lb.
Total weight to lose: _____ lb.
Total weight to lose (_____ lb.) ÷ weight to lose each week (_____ lb.)
= time to achieve target weight: _____ weeks
Weight to lose each week (_____ lb.) x 3,500 calories
= weekly negative caloric balance (cal/week)
Weekly negative caloric balance (_____ cal/week) ÷ 7 days/week
= daily negative caloric balance or _____ cal/day

Remember: keep your weight loss program on schedule. You must achieve the daily negative caloric balance by either decreasing your caloric consumption (eating less) or increasing your caloric expenditure (being more active). A combination of the two strategies will probably be most successful.

You can use the above calculation if your weight loss goal is more than one pound a week. If losing one pound a week feels right to you, then you can figure on decreasing your caloric intake by five hundred calories a day.

The following will be a thirty-day exercise and nutrition log so that you can see your progress on paper. It would be extremely helpful to get a pocket-sized calorie-counting book. If you do not want to do this, just read the label on the side of the food item. It is important to become acquainted with "serving sizes." You may want to use a small scale until you become familiar with what a size looks like.

Most people need a two-thousand-calorie diet to maintain their current weight. So we will use this as our starting point. If you find that you are losing weight too quickly (or slowly), you can adjust this number a couple of hundred calories in either direction.

Remember, when making food choices, your best bet is to incorporate lots of fruits and vegetables, whole grains, and lean meats. Oh, and don't forget your eight eight-ounce glasses of water every day. Congratulations on a new and healthy you, and good luck!

Fit For Life!

Day 1

Breakfast	Calories _____
Snack	Calories _____
Lunch	Calories _____
Dinner	Calories _____
Snack	Calories _____

Total calories for the day   Calories _____

Total number of eight-ounce glasses of water   _____
(minimum of eight glasses)

Total number of minutes of aerobic exercise   _____
(minimum of twenty minutes)

Weight training program for general fitness. Eight-to-ten weight training exercises that focus on major muscle groups done two to three days per week, one to three sets. If you are very ambitious and enjoy strength training, you may do it every day by alternating upper body one day and lower body the next. Keep a record of your accomplishments by marking the exercises done each day.

Exercise		Resistance	Repetitions	Sets
1.	Bench press			
2.	Overhead press			
3.	Lateral pulls			
4.	Lateral raises			
5.	Bicep curls			
6.	Squats			
7.	Toe raises			
8.	Abdominal curls			
9.	Spine extensions			
10.	Neck flexion			

Upper Body Workout		Resistance	Repetitions	Sets
1.	Pec press			
2.	Chest flys			
3.	Biceps curl			
4.	Lateral-side raises			
5.	Triceps toner			
6.	Chest press			

7. Shoulder press   _____
8. Triceps extension   _____
9. One-arm row   _____
10. Push-ups   _____

Lower Body Workout	*Resistance*	*Repetitions*	*Sets*
1. Basic stomach crunch			
2. Basic squats			
3. Basic outer thigh leg lift			
4. Basic inner thigh leg lift			
5. Walking lunges			
6. Calf raises			
7. Oblique crunch			
8. Buttocks firmer			
9. Power lunge			